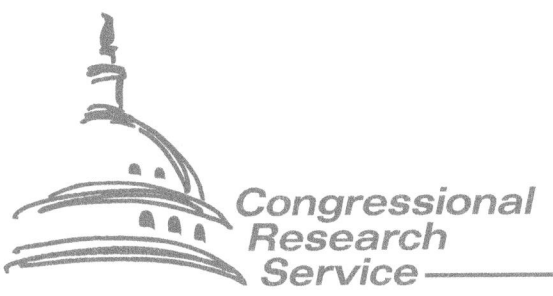 

Health Insurance Exchanges Under the Patient Protection and Affordable Care Act (ACA)

Bernadette Fernandez
Specialist in Health Care Financing

Annie L. Mach
Analyst in Health Care Financing

October 10, 2012

Congressional Research Service
7-5700
www.crs.gov
R42663

CRS Report for Congress
Prepared for Members and Committees of Congress

Summary

The fundamental purpose of a health insurance exchange is to provide a structured marketplace for the sale and purchase of health insurance. The authority and responsibilities of an exchange may vary, depending on statutory or other requirements for its establishment and structure. The Patient Protection and Affordable Care Act (ACA, P.L. 111-148, as amended) requires health insurance exchanges to be established in every state by January 1, 2014. ACA provides certain requirements for the establishment of exchanges, while leaving other choices to be made by the states.

Qualified individuals and small businesses will be able to purchase private health insurance through exchanges. Issuers selling health insurance plans through an exchange will have to follow certain rules, such as meeting the private market reform requirements in ACA. While the fundamental purpose of the exchanges will be to facilitate the offer and purchase of health insurance, nothing in the law prohibits qualified individuals, qualified employers, and insurance carriers from participating in the health insurance market outside of exchanges. Moreover, ACA explicitly states that enrollment in exchanges is voluntary and no individual may be compelled to enroll in exchange coverage.

Exchanges may be established either by the state itself as a "state exchange" or by the Secretary of Health and Human Services (HHS) as a "federally facilitated exchange." All exchanges are required to carry out many of the same functions and adhere to many of the same standards, although there are important differences between the types of exchanges. States will need to declare their intentions to establish their own exchanges by no later than November 16, 2012.

ACA and regulations require exchanges to carry out a number of different functions. The primary functions relate to determining eligibility and enrolling individuals in appropriate plans, plan management, consumer assistance and accountability, and financial management. ACA gives various federal agencies, primarily HHS, responsibilities relating to the general operation of exchanges. Federal agencies are generally responsible for promulgating regulations, creating criteria and systems, and awarding grants to states to help them create and implement exchanges.

A state that is approved to operate its own exchange has a number of operational decisions to make, including decisions related to organizational structure (governmental agency or a nonprofit entity); types of exchanges (separate individual and Small Business Health Options Program (SHOP) exchanges, or a merged exchange); collaboration (a state may independently operate an exchange or enter into contracts with other states); service area (a state may establish one or more subsidiary exchanges in the state if each exchange serves a geographically distinct area and meets certain size requirements); contracted services (an exchange may contract with certain entities to carry out one or more responsibilities of the exchange); and governance (governing board and standards of conduct).

In general, health plans offered through exchanges will provide comprehensive coverage and meet all applicable private market reforms specified in ACA. Most exchange plans will provide coverage for "essential health benefits," at minimum; be subject to certain limits on cost-sharing, including out-of-pocket costs; and meet one of four levels of plan generosity based on actuarial value. To make exchange coverage more affordable, certain individuals will receive premium assistance in the form of federal tax credits. Moreover, some recipients of premium credits may also receive subsidies toward cost-sharing expenses.

This report outlines the required minimum functions of exchanges, and explains how exchanges are expected to be established and administered under ACA. The coverage offered through exchanges is discussed, and the report concludes with a discussion of how exchanges will interact with selected other ACA provisions.

Contents

Introduction 1
ACA Exchanges 2
Establishment of ACA Exchanges 3
    State Exchanges 4
        Operational Structure of a State Exchange 4
        Governance of a State Exchange 5
    Federally Facilitated Exchange 6
What Exchanges Do 7
    Eligibility and Enrollment 7
        Individual Exchange 8
        SHOP Exchange 13
    Plan Management Responsibilities 14
    Consumer Assistance and Accountability 15
    Financial Management 16
Federal Responsibilities for Establishment and Administration of All Exchanges 17
    Federal Oversight 17
    Federal Financial Assistance 18
Coverage Offered through the Exchanges 19
    Coverage Levels and Benefits 19
        Essential Health Benefits 20
        Cost-Sharing Requirements 21
        Levels of Plan Generosity 22
    Exchange Health Plans 23
        Qualified Health Plans 23
        Multi-state Qualified Health Plans 23
        Child-Only Qualified Health Plans 24
        Consumer Operated and Oriented Plans 24
        Catastrophic Plan 25
        Stand-Alone Dental Benefits 26
    Cost Assistance 26
        Premium Tax Credits 26
        Cost-Sharing Subsidies 27
Interaction with Other ACA Provisions 28
    Individual Mandate 28
    Employer Requirements 29
    Reforms to Private Health Insurance Markets 29
    Medicaid 30

Tables

Table 1. Criteria for Determining Eligibility for Enrollment in a QHP 9
Table 2. Criteria for Determining Eligibility for Subsidies Through an Exchange 10

Table 3. Criteria for Determining or Assessing MAGI-Based Eligibility for Enrollment in Medicaid and CHIP 12
Table 4. Criteria for Determining Eligibility for Enrollment in a BHP 13
Table A-1. Selected Upcoming Exchange Implementation Dates 31
Table B-1. Description of Reinsurance, Risk Corridors, and Risk-Adjustment Provisions of ACA 32

Appendixes

Appendix A. Selected Exchange Implementation Dates 31
Appendix B. Risk Mitigation Programs Under ACA 32

Contacts

Author Contact Information... 32

Introduction

A health insurance exchange is a structured marketplace for the sale and purchase of health insurance. "Customers" can include individuals and businesses. The insurance companies ("issuers") that choose to sell their products through an exchange may be required to comply with consumer protections, such as offering insurance to every qualified applicant. Exchanges, however, are not issuers; rather, exchanges contract with issuers who will make insurance products available for purchase through exchanges. Essentially, exchanges are designed to bring together buyers and sellers of insurance, with the goal of increasing access to coverage.

This rather broad definition allows for a great deal of latitude, and therefore variance, in the number and scope of responsibilities covered in a particular exchange. For example, the role of an exchange may be more or less administrative: facilitating the sale and purchase of health insurance. An administrative-only exchange may function similar to websites that allow individuals to find airline travel options and purchase tickets (e.g., Kayak). Such an approach does not necessarily change or establish standards for the products being sold (whether they are health plans or airline tickets), or limit the types of buyers and sellers participating in the exchange, beyond what already exists in the private market. An example of a minimalist health insurance exchange is the Utah Health Exchange. Essentially, Utah's exchange is an internet portal that is "designed to connect consumers to the information they need to make informed health care choices, and in the case of health insurance, to execute that choice electronically."[1]

At the other end of the spectrum, an exchange may have multiple functions beyond the role of insurance marketplace. For instance, an exchange may be responsible for implementing regulatory standards, such as requiring standardization of all products offered through it or imposing requirements on exchange participants. An exchange may be responsible for determining eligibility for exchange plans and government-provided subsidies. An example of a more regulatory-oriented exchange is the Health Connector ("Connector") in Massachusetts. Similar to Utah's exchange, the Connector provides an online tool to allow consumers and others to find commercial health insurance options available to them. In addition, the Connector also manages a publicly subsidized coverage program for low-income state residents, and offers certificates to exempt individuals from the state's individual mandate, among other duties.[2]

An exchange may occupy a physical location and/or be virtual (i.e., performing its functions on the Internet). It may be governed by a public agency, a private entity, or a hybrid organization. The insurance options offered through an exchange may also vary across insurance markets[3] and plan types. Nonetheless, while the authority and responsibilities of an exchange may vary, its fundamental purpose is to provide a venue where insurance companies may sell their insurance products and purchasers can compare and choose from multiple options available to them. Thus an exchange allows for "one-stop shopping" with respect to health insurance.

---

[1] "Utah Health Exchange," http://www.exchange.utah.gov/about-the-exchange.

[2] "Health Connector," https://www.mahealthconnector.org/portal/site/connector.

[3] The private health insurance market is made up of three segments—the large group, small group and nongroup (individual) markets. The nongroup market refers to insurance policies offered to individuals and families buying insurance on their own. Group insurance refers to health plans offered through a plan sponsor, typically an employer.

The exchange concept was included in the Patient Protection and Affordable Care Act (ACA, P.L. 111-148, as amended), as a means to increase access to health insurance. While ACA places many restrictions on the design and function of exchanges, the law also leaves many operational decisions to the states. Such flexibility will likely lead to variation in exchange models across the states. For example, a state may decide to operate an exchange by itself, establish an exchange in partnership with the federal government, or leave this work entirely to the federal government. The deadlines for making such complex decisions are approaching quickly. By November 16, 2012, states must declare whether or not they will assume the responsibility for establishing exchanges. The initial open enrollment period will begin on October 1, 2013, and exchanges are to be operational and offering coverage on January 1, 2014.

This report looks at the requirements for exchanges established in ACA and provides information on the requirements and choices available to states for the establishment, functions, financial responsibilities, and coverage of the ACA exchanges. It also includes a brief discussion of the interactions between exchanges and other provisions in the law.

ACA Exchanges

ACA intends exchanges to be marketplaces where qualified individuals and small businesses can "shop" for private health insurance coverage.[4] The coverage offered through exchanges will be comprehensive[5] and meet all applicable private market reforms[6] specified in ACA. Such plans offered through the exchanges will be certified as "qualified health plans" or QHPs.[7]

ACA explicitly states that enrollment in exchanges is voluntary and no individual may be compelled to enroll in exchange coverage.[8] While the main purpose of the exchanges will be to facilitate the offer and purchase of health insurance, nothing in the ACA prohibits qualified individuals, qualified small businesses, and insurance carriers from participating in the health insurance market outside of exchanges.[9]

For individuals seeking coverage, exchanges will not only create marketplaces where qualified individuals can purchase QHPs in the nongroup (individual) market, but exchanges will also

---

[4] Before 2016, states will have the option to define "small employers" either as those with 100 or fewer employees or 50 or fewer employees. Beginning in 2016, small employers will be defined as those with 100 or fewer employees. Beginning in 2017, states may allow large employers to obtain coverage through an exchange (but will not be required to do so).

[5] With the exception of stand-alone dental plans that are allowed to be offered in the exchanges.

[6] For additional information about ACA's private market reforms, see CRS Report R42069, *Private Health Insurance Market Reforms in the Patient Protection and Affordable Care Act (ACA)*, by Annie L. Mach and Bernadette Fernandez.

[7] As discussed in the "Plan Management Responsibilities" section of this report, a plan has to meet certain statutory requirements to be certified as a QHP. Certain plans offered through exchanges (e.g., stand-alone dental plans) do not necessarily meet all of the criteria to be certified as a QHP; however, the plans are required to meet some criteria and are considered QHPs for the purpose of how the exchange interacts with the plan. For example, while a stand-alone dental plan cannot meet criteria related to benefits to qualify as a QHP (because the plan only offers dental benefits), a stand-alone dental plan is still required to meet the QHP standard to annually provide benefit and rate information to the exchange.

[8] §1312(d)(3)(B) of ACA.

[9] §1312(d)(1) of ACA.

assist individuals with obtaining federally subsidized premium and cost-sharing assistance to help low to middle income individuals offset the cost of both purchasing and using health insurance. Exchanges will also screen individuals for eligibility for certain public insurance programs (e.g., Medicaid) and connect them with appropriate agencies.

Small businesses seeking coverage for their employees will be able to use the small business health options program (SHOP) exchange. The SHOP exchange is designed to assist qualified small employers and their employees with the purchase of QHPs offered in the small group market. Qualified small employers will be able to select QHPs available in the SHOP to offer to their employees, and they will be able to set the amount they will contribute to QHP premiums.

ACA requires exchanges to be established in every state by January 1, 2014. Exchanges must be established by the state itself or by the Secretary of Health and Human Services (HHS),[10] and they must carry out the general functions described above for both individuals and small businesses. Additionally, exchanges will be expected to perform a number of other functions relating to managing the QHPs offered through the exchanges and assisting individuals and small businesses in accessing and obtaining coverage.

Establishment of ACA Exchanges

ACA provides general direction regarding the establishment and administration of an exchange. ACA is supplemented by the final regulation on the establishment of exchanges and other guidance produced by federal agencies, particularly HHS.[11] Taken together, these documents set forth some requirements and minimum standards that various stakeholders—including consumers, states, issuers, and employers—must meet to be part of or to participate in an exchange.

One factor that could influence a number of determinations related to how an exchange is implemented is whether the exchange is established by a state or HHS. States have the option of establishing their own exchanges ("state exchange") as a governmental agency or a non-profit entity. If a state wants to operate its own exchange beginning January 1, 2014, it must submit required documents no later than November 16, 2012 for the exchange to be approved by HHS by January 1, 2013.[12]

If a state's exchange is not approved, or if a state chooses not to establish its own exchange, the HHS Secretary has the authority to establish and operate an exchange in that state directly, or through an agreement with a non-profit entity.[13] In a "federally-facilitated exchange," HHS will carry out all functions of the exchange and have authority over the exchange. HHS gives states the option to enter into a hybrid type of exchange—somewhere between a state exchange and a federally facilitated exchange. This option is referred to as a "partnership" with a federally facilitated exchange, whereby certain state-designed and operated functions are combined with

---

[10] §§ 1311(b) and 1321(c) of ACA.

[11] 77 *Federal Register* 18310, March 27, 2012.

[12] §1311(b) of ACA. In August 2012, HHS released the "Blueprint for Approval of Affordable State-based and State Partnership Insurance Exchanges," which states are required to submit by November 16, 2012, to meet the 2013 approval date. The Blueprint is available at http://cciio.cms.gov/resources/files/hie-blueprint-081312.pdf.

[13] §1321(c) of ACA.

federally designed and operated functions. While HHS and states share responsibility for carrying out functions in partnerships within federally facilitated exchanges, HHS retains authority over these exchanges.[14]

Regardless of whether an exchange is established by a state or the federal government, the initial open enrollment period for an exchange will be October 1, 2013 through March 31, 2014. Exchanges must begin offering coverage to qualified individuals and small businesses on January 1, 2014.[15]

State Exchanges

The HHS Secretary must approve the operation of a state exchange if it meets the following standards:

- the exchange is able to carry out the required functions of the exchange as established in the law and regulation, which include making QHPs available to qualified individuals and qualified employers;
- the exchange is capable of carrying out the information reporting requirements related to sharing information with the federal government in order to determine an individual's eligibility for a premium tax credit;[16] and
- either the entire geographic area of the state is covered in the exchange or the state has established multiple exchanges that cover the entire geographic area of the state.[17]

A state exchange is responsible for creating and implementing its structure and governing system according to the guidelines outlined in the statute and regulations, as discussed below.

Operational Structure of a State Exchange

A state that is approved to establish its own exchange has a number of decisions to make regarding the exchange's operational structure. A state must determine whether its exchange will be a governmental agency or a non-profit established by the state. The terms "governmental" and "non-profit established by the state," have not been defined; instead, it seems these terms are subject to state interpretation.[18]

---

[14] 77 *Federal Register* 18310, March 27, 2012. The law also requires that the HHS Secretary creates a process whereby states that were operating exchanges before January 1, 2010 can receive assistance from federal agencies to bring their exchanges into compliance with the requirements under ACA (§1322(e) of ACA).

[15] Selected exchange implementation dates are shown in **Table A-1**. It should be noted that the final rule on exchange establishment (77 *Federal Register* 18310, March 27, 2012) provides for ways in which states can change the type of exchange established in the state. For example, if a state chooses not to establish an exchange for 2014, it still may elect to do so in the future.

[16] For a comprehensive discussion of the premium tax credits, see CRS Report R41137, *Health Insurance Premium Credits in the Patient Protection and Affordable Care Act (ACA)*, by Bernadette Fernandez and Thomas Gabe.

[17] 77 *Federal Register* 18310, March 27, 2012.

[18] In responding to requests for clarification regarding what would be considered "governmental," HHS has said that it will not offer further clarification of "governmental" in deference to existing state classifications. HHS has not commented on the definition of a non-profit established by a state.

A state can choose to independently operate an exchange, or a state can enter into contracts with other states (regardless of whether the states are contiguous) to operate a regional exchange.[19] States can also establish one or more subsidiary exchanges in the state if each exchange serves a geographically distinct area and if the area served by each exchange meets the geographic size requirement established in the law.[20] In other words, while states have a great deal of leeway in establishing how the exchange is divided up geographically, they must serve the entire population in their state. Furthermore, regional exchanges and subsidiary exchanges must meet all exchange requirements.

A state exchange must operate both the individual and SHOP exchanges, but a state can either merge the exchanges and operate both under the same administrative and governance structures, or elect to create separate administrative and governance structures for the individual and SHOP exchanges.[21] Additionally, regional and subsidiary exchanges must perform the functions of a SHOP exchange. If an exchange chooses to operate an individual exchange and a SHOP exchange under two different governance and administrative structures, a SHOP exchange must cover the same geographic area as the regional or subsidiary individual exchange.[22]

States also have the authority to allow a state exchange to contract with the entities described below to carry out one or more responsibilities of the exchange.[23] States can grant this authority to state exchanges independent of whether an exchange is a governmental agency or a non-profit established by the state. For example, a state exchange that is a non-profit established by the state could contract with a state agency that meets the criteria below to carry out certain consumer assistance functions for the exchange.

A state exchange may contract with

- an entity, including a state agency other than a Medicaid agency, incorporated under and subject to the laws of at least one state, that has demonstrated experience on a state or regional basis in the individual and small group health insurance markets and in benefits coverage, but is not an issuer; and/or
- a state Medicaid agency.

Governance of a State Exchange

Generally, a state exchange must have a governing board that meets certain requirements; the board must[24]

- be administered under a publicly adopted operating charter or by-laws;

---

[19] §1311(f)(1) of ACA. Each state participating in the regional exchange must permit the operation of the regional exchange, and the HHS Secretary has to approve the regional exchange before it can begin operation.

[20] §1311(f)(2) of ACA. The area served by a subsidiary exchange must be at least as large as a rating area approved by the HHS Secretary for purposes described in §2701 of the Public Health Service Act (PHSA).

[21] §1311(b)(2) of ACA.

[22] 77 *Federal Register* 18310, March 27, 2012.

[23] §1311(f)(3) of ACA and 77 *Federal Register* 18310, March 27, 2012. If an exchange contracts out any function of the exchange, the exchange is responsible for ensuring that the contracted entity meets all federal requirements related to the function.

[24] 77 *Federal Register* 18310, March 27, 2012.

- hold regular meetings that are open to the public and announced in advance;
- ensure that the board's membership includes at least one voting member who is a consumer representative and is not made up of a majority of voting representatives with conflicts of interest (e.g., representatives of issuers); and
- ensure that a majority of the voting members on its governing board have relevant experience in the health care field (e.g., in health benefits administration, or in public health).

In addition, a state exchange is required to have in place and make publicly available a set of governance principles that include ethics, conflict of interest standards, transparency and accounting standards, and standards related to disclosure of financial interests. A state exchange must also implement procedures as to how members of the governing board will disclose any financial interests. The state exchange's governance principles are subject to periodic review by HHS.[25]

Federally Facilitated Exchange

If a state chooses not to operate its own exchange, or if a state does not have approval to operate its own exchange as of January 1, 2013, the HHS Secretary is required to establish a "federally-facilitated exchange" in the state.[26] A federally facilitated exchange can be implemented by HHS alone, or a state can enter into a "partnership" with a federally facilitated exchange, combining state-designed and operated functions with federally designed and operated functions.[27] Partnerships are considered a "subset" of federally facilitated exchanges, indicating that HHS has authority over partnerships in federally facilitated exchanges.[28]

The final rule on the establishment of exchanges does not include provisions specific to federally facilitated exchanges (instead saying that information for these exchanges will be provided in future guidance). However, the final rule does indicate that federally facilitated exchanges are required to carry-out many of the same functions as state exchanges. Additionally, federally facilitated exchanges and state exchanges must adhere to many of the same standards outlined in ACA and the final rule. For example, state exchanges and federally facilitated exchanges are both required to offer the same tools to help consumers access an exchange and assess their plan options through an exchange.

Although there are no specific regulations related to federally facilitated exchanges, HHS has published some *guidance*, which generally describes how HHS will operate federally facilitated exchanges within the framework established by ACA and the final rule.[29] This guidance includes

---

[25] Ibid.

[26] §1321(c) of ACA.

[27] The partnership model is discussed in an HHS fact sheet published September 19, 2011, available at http://www.healthcare.gov/news/factsheets/2011/09/exchanges09192011a.html. The partnership model and the federally facilitated exchange model are both discussed in the final rule on establishment of exchanges (77 *Federal Register* 18310, March 27, 2012). Finally, more information is provided about federally facilitated exchanges, including partnerships, in guidance released May 16, 2012, available at http://cciio.cms.gov/resources/files/FFE_Guidance_FINAL_VERSION_051612.pdf.

[28] 77 *Federal Register* 18310, March 27, 2012.

[29] Center for Consumer Information and Insurance Oversight, *General Guidance on Federally-facilitated Exchanges*, May 16, 2012, http://cciio.cms.gov/resources/files/FFE_Guidance_FINAL_VERSION_051612.pdf.

information such as descriptions of a state's potential responsibilities if the state decides to enter into a partnership with a federally facilitated exchange. Further guidance related to federally facilitated exchanges is expected.

What Exchanges Do

Exchanges are required to carry out a number of different functions, including determining eligibility and enrolling individuals in appropriate plans; conducting plan management activities; assisting consumers, ensuring plan accountability; and providing financial management.[30] These functions are not necessarily exhaustive of exchange responsibilities; rather, this section is intended to provide a general overview of an exchange's responsibilities. Unless otherwise noted, both state and federally facilitated exchanges are required to carry out the functions described in this section. Additionally, some responsibilities may be different for individual exchanges and SHOP exchanges, so the following discussion provides information for both.

Eligibility and Enrollment

Exchanges are responsible for a variety of functions related to determining an applicant's eligibility (whether an individual's or an employer's) for various plans/programs and for enrolling eligible applicants into those plans/programs. With these eligibility and enrollment responsibilities come the responsibility to verify the information received from applicants and to re-determine eligibility as necessary. Exchanges are expected to have secure electronic databases in place that support exchanges' eligibility and enrollment responsibilities by allowing information to be shared among state and federal agencies.[31] An exchange's responsibilities to determine eligibility and to enroll eligible individuals are different, but related, for the individual exchange and the SHOP exchange (for small business employees).

Flexibility Related to Eligibility and Enrollment Systems

ACA intends to create a seamless eligibility and enrollment system for individuals seeking health insurance coverage in the nongroup market and/or through public programs (e.g., Medicaid). The system would allow individuals to fill out a single application that collects the information necessary to screen the individual for multiple types of coverage and financial assistance. The system would then facilitate the enrollment of the individual in the appropriate plan/program.

States have some flexibility in designing and implementing this streamlined system. The flexibility is related to how eligibility and enrollment responsibilities will be shared among entities, including individual exchanges. ACA requires that the system is able to determine an applicant's eligibility for enrollment in a QHP[32] and for insurance affordability programs (IAP),[33] which include Medicaid, the State Children's Health Insurance Program (CHIP), the Basic Health Program (BHP),[34] advanced payment of premium tax credits, and cost-sharing reductions.

---

[30] The framework for this section is adapted from a report co-authored by Deborah Bachrach and Patricia Boozang, titled, "Federally-Facilitated Exchanges and the Continuum of State Options," available at http://www.nasi.org/research/2011/federally-facilitated-exchanges-continuum-state-options.

[31] §§ 1413 and 1561 of ACA. The most recent guidance (May 2011) produced by Centers for Medicare & Medicaid Services (CMS) addressing the electronic databases is available at http://www.medicaid.gov/Medicaid-CHIP-Program-Information/By-Topics/Data-and-Systems/Downloads/exchangemedicaiditguidance.pdf.

[32] For more information about QHPs offered through an exchange, see the "Qualified Health Plans" section of this report.

[33] The term and definition of "insurance affordability programs" is adopted from a definition in the final rule on exchange establishment (77 *Federal Register* 18310, March 27, 2012).

> ACA and regulations allow different entities to participate in the eligibility and enrollment system. For example, the system can be designed to enable one entity (e.g., the individual exchange) to determine eligibility for and effectuate enrollment in QHPs and all IAPs. Alternatively, the system can be designed so that one state agency determines eligibility for one IAP (i.e., the state's Medicaid agency determines Medicaid eligibility) while another entity or other entities determine eligibility for other plans/programs.
>
> Descriptions of the potential variations in eligibility and enrollment systems that may occur as a result of this flexibility are beyond the scope of this report. However, it is important to note that this section generally describes how an individual exchange would handle its eligibility and enrollment functions *if it were to carry out the functions*. The summaries of eligibility requirements for enrollment in plans/programs described in **Table 1**, **Table 2**, **Table 3**, and **Table 4** are the same regardless of which entity determines eligibility.

Individual Exchange

To determine eligibility, an individual exchange must use a single, streamlined application to collect information from an applicant and verify that information according to procedures identified in regulation. For example, an individual exchange is expected to verify an applicant's social security number by transmitting the number to HHS, which will consult the Social Security Administration and the Department of Homeland Security, as needed, to verify the number.[35]

An individual exchange is expected to re-determine an enrollee's eligibility if the individual exchange receives and verifies new information relating to the enrollee. This information can come from the enrollee, as enrollees are required to report any change with respect to eligibility standards within 30 days of the change, or it can come from information the individual exchange finds through its required periodic examination of available information that might affect eligibility (e.g., whether an enrollee has died). An individual exchange is also expected to re-determine or re-assess the eligibility of all enrollees on an annual basis. However, re-determinations and re-assessments due to changes in status do not fully satisfy the requirement for annual re-determinations and re-assessments.[36]

Eligibility for Enrollment in a QHP

An individual exchange is required to *determine* an applicant's eligibility for enrollment in a QHP. If an applicant is determined eligible for a QHP, the individual exchange is expected to facilitate the applicant's enrollment into the QHP selected by the individual. **Table 1** shows the criteria an individual exchange must use to determine eligibility for enrollment in a QHP.

(...continued)

[34] §1331 of ACA requires the HHS Secretary to create a basic health program (BHP), which is a health insurance program for low-income individuals who are not eligible for Medicaid, and is offered in lieu of eligible individuals obtaining coverage through an exchange. States have the option to implement the BHP, and therefore, exchanges will interact with BHPs in only those states that choose to implement a BHP.

[35] 77 *Federal Register* 18310, March 27, 2012.

[36] Ibid.

Table 1. Criteria for Determining Eligibility for Enrollment in a QHP

	An individual exchange must determine an applicant eligible for a QHP if the applicant meets the following criteria:
Enrollment in a QHP	• Citizen, national, or noncitizen who is lawfully present in the United States[a] • Not incarcerated, other than pending the disposition of charges • Meets applicable state residency standards

Source: CRS analysis of ACA (as amended) and 77 *Federal Register* 18310, March 27, 2012.

a. Only lawful residents may obtain exchange coverage; unauthorized aliens will be prohibited from obtaining coverage through an exchange, even if they could pay the entire premium without a subsidy.

Eligibility for Premium Tax Credits and Cost-Sharing Subsidies

Certain individuals who purchase a QHP through an individual exchange will be eligible for financial assistance to help them off-set the cost of the coverage and to defray some costs associated with using health services. ACA provides assistance, for the purchase of exchange coverage, in the form of premium tax credits. (A tax credit is a reduction that is applied to the amount an individual (or family) owes, if any, when filing income taxes.) Premium tax credits are advanceable, meaning instead of having to wait until after the end of the tax year to receive the credit, the individual may receive the payments in advance to coincide with when insurance premiums are due (usually on a monthly basis).

In addition to the premium tax credits, ACA provides cost-sharing subsides to certain individuals to help them pay costs related to the use of health services. (Cost-sharing generally refers to costs that an individual must pay when using services that are covered under the health plan that the person is enrolled in; common forms of cost-sharing include copayments and deductibles.) Both premium tax credits and cost-sharing subsidies are discussed later in this report under the section "Cost Assistance."

Because the premium tax credits are advanceable, it will be necessary to determine an individual's eligibility for the credits at the time the individual applies for coverage through an exchange. In regard to advanced payment of premium tax credits, an individual exchange may either *determine* an applicant's eligibility directly or *implement a determination* of eligibility made by HHS.[37] Determining eligibility directly is similar to determining eligibility for QHPs; the individual exchange reviews an applicant's information and makes a determination of eligibility. If an individual exchange chooses to determine an applicant's eligibility for advance payment of premium tax credits, the exchange must calculate the amount of the advance payment in accordance with section 36B of the Internal Revenue Code. An individual exchange may only provide the advance payment if the applicant meets the eligibility criteria (see **Table 2**).

Similarly, an individual exchange may either directly determine eligibility for cost-sharing subsidies, or it may implement a determination made by HHS. If an individual exchange chooses to determine an applicant's eligibility for cost-sharing subsidies, the exchange must do so according to the criteria outlined in **Table 2**.

---

[37] These provisions were included as "interim final" rather than in the final rule on exchange establishment (77 *Federal Register* 18310, March 27, 2012), and comments were accepted on both provisions through May 11, 2012. The preamble of the final rule indicates that further guidance on these provisions is forthcoming.

If an individual exchange decides *not* to directly determine eligibility for advanced payment of premium tax credits or *not* to directly determine eligibility for cost-sharing subsidies but rather implements HHS determinations, then an individual exchange is expected to transmit all collected and verified information to HHS. The individual exchange does not make a recommendation in this process; rather, the individual exchange shares information with HHS and then is expected to adhere to the determination of eligibility made by HHS.[38]

Table 2. Criteria for Determining Eligibility for Subsidies Through an Exchange

An exchange or HHS may determine an applicant eligible for the subsidies below according to the following criteria:	
Advanced payment of premium tax credits	• Meets the criteria for eligibility for enrollment in a QHP through an exchange[a]
	• Not eligible for minimum essential coverage (other than through the individual health insurance market)[b]
	• Is part of a tax-filing unit
	• Is enrolled in a QHP offered through an exchange
	• Has household income that either
	• is between 100% and 400% FPL; or
	• is not greater than 100% FPL and is an alien lawfully present (but not eligible for Medicaid because of duration of U.S. residency)[d]
Cost-sharing subsidies	• Meets the criteria for eligibility for enrollment in a QHP through an exchange
	• Meets the criteria for eligibility for advance payment of premium tax credits
	• Is enrolled in a silver plan through an exchange[d]
	• Has household income between 100% and 400% FPL[e]

Source: CRS analysis of ACA (as amended) and 77 Federal Register 18310, March 27, 2012.

a. These criteria are detailed in **Table 1**.

b. The definition of minimum essential coverage is discussed in CRS Report R41331, *Individual Mandate and Related Information Requirements under ACA*, by Janemarie Mulvey and Hinda Chaikind.

c. The Personal Responsibility and Work Opportunity Reconciliation Act of 1996 (P.L. 104-193) determined that most individuals who are not citizens but are lawfully present in the United States are barred from Medicaid for the first five years that they are in the United States.

d. A description of the different tiers of coverage offered through an exchange is included in the "Coverage Levels and Benefits" section of this report.

e. The cost-sharing subsidies reduces the annual caps on out-of-pocket expenses for individuals with income between 100% and 400% FPL. Additionally, ACA requires QHP issuers to further reduce cost-sharing requirements for individuals with income between 100% and 250% FPL. For more information, see CRS Report R41137, *Health Insurance Premium Credits in the Patient Protection and Affordable Care Act (ACA)*, by Bernadette Fernandez and Thomas Gabe.

---

[38] The eligibility criteria for advance payment of premium tax credits and cost-sharing subsidies are the same regardless of whether an individual exchange makes the determination or HHS makes the determination.

Eligibility for Medicaid and CHIP

An individual exchange may either *determine* or *assess* an applicant's eligibility for enrollment in Medicaid and/or CHIP. If an individual exchange *determines* eligibility for Medicaid and/or CHIP, then the individual exchange is also responsible for the enrollment of eligible applicants. Once an applicant has been determined eligible, the individual exchange must transmit the applicant's information to the state Medicaid or CHIP agency, thus effectuating enrollment.

An individual exchange may only *assess* eligibility for Medicaid/CHIP. If an applicant is assessed eligible for a program the individual exchange is required to transmit all collected and verified information to the state Medicaid or CHIP agency to enable the agency to make a final determination of the applicant's eligibility. In this case, the exchange is only making a recommendation and sharing information with the appropriate agency; it is not responsible for making a final determination of eligibility. The individual exchange is expected to adhere to the final determination made by the agency.

The final rule on Medicaid eligibility changes under ACA indicates that the state Medicaid and/or CHIP agency will decide whether an individual exchange will determine or assess eligibility for its program(s).[39] Additionally, the rule clarifies that some individuals have financial eligibility for Medicaid based on modified adjusted gross income (MAGI), while others do not have financial eligibility based on MAGI.[40] The rule provides that a state's Medicaid agency can separately decide on the individual exchange's role in determining or assessing Medicaid eligibility for MAGI and non-MAGI populations. **Table 3** shows criteria an individual exchange must use to determine or assess eligibility for individuals whose financial eligibility is based on MAGI. It is beyond the scope of this report to detail the criteria used to determine or assess eligibility for individuals whose financial eligibility is not based on MAGI.

---

[39] 77 *Federal Register* 17144, March 23, 2012.

[40] On June 28, 2012, the United States Supreme Court issued its decision in *National Federation of Independent Business v. Sebelius*. The Court held that the federal government cannot terminate current Medicaid program federal matching funds if a state refuses to expand its Medicaid program to include non-elderly, non-pregnant adults under 133% of the federal poverty level. If a state accepts the new ACA Medicaid expansion funds, it must abide by the new expansion coverage rules, but, based on the Court's opinion, it appears that a state can refuse to participate in the expansion without losing any of its current federal Medicaid matching funds. This decision did not affect the ACA requirement that modified adjusted gross income (MAGI) would be the new income test for most of Medicaid's covered populations beginning in 2014. For a legal analysis of the Court's decision on Medicaid, see CRS General Distribution Memorandum, *Selected Issues Related to the Effect of NFIB v. Sebelius on the Medicaid Expansion Requirements in Section 2001 of the Affordable Care Act*, by Kathleen S. Swendiman and Evelyne P. Baumrucker. For a comprehensive discussion about MAGI and ACA, see CRS Report R41997, *Definition of Income in ACA for Certain Medicaid Provisions and Premium Credits*, coordinated by Janemarie Mulvey.

Table 3. Criteria for Determining or Assessing MAGI-Based Eligibility for Enrollment in Medicaid and CHIP

An individual exchange may determine an applicant eligible or assess an applicant's eligibility for MAGI-based Medicaid and CHIP according to the following criteria:		
	Determination	**Assessment**
Enrollment in Medicaid	• Meets the non-financial criteria for Medicaid for populations whose eligibility is based on modified adjusted gross income (MAGI)[a] • Has a household income that is at or below the applicable Medicaid MAGI-based income standard • Is either a pregnant woman, under age 19, a parent or caretaker of a dependent child, or is under age 65 and not entitled to or enrolled in Medicare Parts A or B	• Makes the assessment based on the applicable Medicaid MAGI-based income standards and citizenship and immigration status, using verification rules and procedures consistent with Medicaid statute, regardless of how such standards are implemented by the state Medicaid agency • Must adhere to state Medicaid agency's final determination of applicant's eligibility
Enrollment in CHIP	• Meets the requirements for children to enroll in CHIP[b] • Has a household income at or below the applicable CHIP MAGI-based income standard	• Makes the assessment based on the applicable CHIP MAGI-based income standards and citizenship and immigration status, using verification rules and procedures consistent with CHIP statute, regardless of how such standards are implemented by the state CHIP agency • Must adhere to state CHIP agency's final determination of applicant's eligibility

Source: CRS analysis of ACA (as amended) and 77 *Federal Register* 18310, March 27, 2012.

a. For information about populations whose Medicaid eligibility is, in part, based on MAGI-based income, see CRS Report R41210, *Medicaid and the State Children's Health Insurance Program (CHIP) Provisions in ACA: Summary and Timeline*, by Evelyne P. Baumrucker et al.

b. For more information about children's eligibility for CHIP, see CRS Report R40444, *State Children's Health Insurance Program (CHIP): A Brief Overview*, by Elicia J. Herz and Evelyne P. Baumrucker.

Eligibility for Enrollment in a BHP

The Basic Health Program (BHP) is a health insurance program for low-income individuals who are not eligible for Medicaid, and is offered in lieu of eligible individuals obtaining coverage through an exchange. States have the option to implement the BHP, and therefore, exchanges will interact with BHPs in only those states that choose to implement a BHP.

If a state chooses to establish a BHP, an individual exchange is expected to *determine* an applicant's eligibility for a BHP, and facilitate the applicant's enrollment in the program. **Table 4** shows the criteria an individual exchange must use to determine eligibility for enrollment in a BHP.

Table 4. Criteria for Determining Eligibility for Enrollment in a BHP

	An individual exchange must determine an applicant eligible for a BHP if the applicant meets the following criteria:

Enrollment in the Basic Health Program (BHP)	• Resident of a state and not eligible for the state's Medicaid program
	• Not eligible for minimum essential coverage or is eligible for employer-sponsored insurance (ESI) that is not affordable[a]
	• Has not attained age 65 at the beginning of the plan year
	• Has household income that either
	    • exceeds 133% of the federal poverty level (FPL) but does not exceed 200% FPL; or
	    • is not greater than 133% FPL and is an alien lawfully present (but not eligible for Medicaid because of duration of U.S. residency)[b]

Source: CRS analysis of ACA (as amended) and 77 *Federal Register* 18310, March 27, 2012.

a. The definition of minimum essential coverage is discussed in CRS Report R41331, *Individual Mandate and Related Information Requirements under ACA*, by Janemarie Mulvey and Hinda Chaikind. ACA considers employer coverage "unaffordable" if the employee's contribution toward the employer's lowest-cost self-only premium exceeds 9.5% of household income.

b. The Personal Responsibility and Work Opportunity Reconciliation Act of 1996 (P.L. 104-193) determined that most individuals who are not citizens but are lawfully present in the United States are barred from Medicaid for the first five years that they are in the United States.

SHOP Exchange

As the exchange for small businesses, the SHOP has responsibilities similar to the individual exchange in that the SHOP is also responsible for collecting and verifying information from employers and employees (both considered applicants), determining eligibility, and facilitating enrollment. An employer and each of its employees seeking coverage must submit an application to the SHOP. The SHOP must process the applications, and if the employer and employees are determined eligible, the SHOP must facilitate the enrollment of qualified employees into QHPs offered through the SHOP.

A qualified employee is an employee who receives an offer of coverage from a qualified employer. A qualified employer is a small group employer[41] that elects to make, at a minimum, all full-time employees eligible for one or more QHPs offered in the small group market through an exchange, and has its principal business in the exchange service area or offers coverage to each eligible employee through the SHOP serving the employee's worksite.[42]

The SHOP is required to verify applicants' eligibility as outlined in regulation.[43] The SHOP must permit an employer to purchase coverage for employees at any time during the year, but the employer's plan must consist of a 12-month period beginning with the employer's effective date

---

[41] Before 2016, states will have the option to define "small employers" either as those with 100 or fewer employees or 50 or fewer employees. Beginning in 2016, small employers will be defined as those with 100 or fewer employees.

[42] Beginning in 2017, a state may also allow an issuer of coverage in the large group market to offer QHPs in the large group market through an exchange. If that is the case, then a qualified employer would also include an employer in the large group market.

[43] 77 *Federal Register* 18310, March 27, 2012.

of coverage. Employees must adhere to annual open enrollment periods as determined by the SHOP, with special allowances for newly qualified employees.

Employers are not required to offer all the plans in an exchange to their employees. The SHOP must allow an employer to limit the selection of plans.[44] An employer who uses the SHOP is not required to contribute to employees' premiums; additionally, neither ACA nor regulations specify whether a SHOP can require a minimum contribution from employers.[45]

Plan Management Responsibilities

Exchanges are required to ensure that QHPs are certified.[46] An exchange may certify a plan as a QHP if the plan meets the required minimum criteria and if the exchange determines that it is in the best interest of qualified individuals and employers to have such a plan available.[47] The minimum certification criteria outlined in ACA and further defined through regulation include requirements related to marketing, choice of providers, plan networks, accreditation,[48] and other features.[49]

In addition to certifying QHPs, an exchange must establish processes for recertification and decertification of QHPs. The recertification process, at a minimum, must include a review of the general certification criteria and must be completed on or before September 15 of the applicable calendar year. The decertification process must, at a minimum, include the following requirements: the ability for an exchange to decertify a plan at any time if the exchange determines that the QHP no longer meets the certification requirements; an exchange must establish a process for the appeal of a decertification; and an exchange must provide a notice of the decertification to all affected parties, including the QHP issuer, the exchange enrollees, HHS, and the state insurance department.

An exchange has additional plan management functions. For example, the exchange must require plans seeking certification as QHPs to submit justification for premium increases before it takes effect, and the plans will have to post the information about their premium increases on their websites.[50] Also, the HHS Secretary is required to create a system that rates QHPs on the basis of

---

[44] Ibid. If a state merges its individual and small group risk pools, as is allowed under §1312(c)(3) of ACA, then the SHOP may permit an employee to enroll in any QHP (including one offered in the individual market), as long as the QHP meets certain requirements for small group market plans.

[45] This information was confirmed through correspondence with analysts from the Center for Consumer Information and Insurance Oversight (CCIIO) in September 2012.

[46] §1311(d)(4)(A) of ACA.

[47] Except that, according to §1311(e)(1)(B) of ACA, the exchange may not exclude a plan because it is a fee-for-service plan, through the imposition of price controls, or on the basis that the plan provides treatments necessary to prevent patients' deaths in circumstances the exchange determines are inappropriate or too costly.

[48] In the final regulation on entities for the accreditation of exchange plans, HHS stated that the National Committee for Quality Assurance and URAC (formerly known as the Utilization Review Accreditation Commission) would serve as accrediting entities during the first phase of the accrediting process. HHS will consider other accrediting bodies and individual states at a later time. 77 *Federal Register* 42662, July 20, 2012.

[49] §1311(c)(1) of ACA and 77 *Federal Register* 18310, March 27, 2012.

[50] §1311(e)(2) of ACA.

relative quality and price. An exchange is expected to assign a rating to each QHP according to the HHS Secretary's criteria and provide the quality rating information through its website.[51]

Consumer Assistance and Accountability

Exchanges have a number of responsibilities related to assisting consumers in accessing and obtaining coverage, including providing tools to help consumers access the exchange, helping consumers determine which plan or program to enroll in, and helping consumers determine their potential financial responsibility for a QHP offered through an exchange.[52] Additionally, exchanges are expected to adhere to accountability practices to increase an exchange's transparency.

The following are some of an exchange's responsibilities related to assisting consumers and being accountable to stakeholders, including consumers. An exchange must

- Provide for operation of a toll-free telephone hotline that addresses the needs of consumers requesting assistance and informs individuals with disabilities and limited English proficiency of the availability of services to assist them.

- Maintain a website which, among other things, provides standardized comparative information on each QHP available through the exchange and allows qualified individuals to select a QHP in which to enroll.[53]

- Make available an electronic calculator (through its website) that facilitates the comparison of available QHPs (including the impact of any advance payments of tax credits and cost-sharing subsidies in the individual exchange and the impact of any employer contribution in the SHOP exchange).

- Conduct outreach and education activities that will educate consumers about the exchange and insurance affordability programs (IAPs) to encourage participation.[54]

- Establish a Navigator program with grants to eligible individuals and entities to provide information about the exchange and help individuals select a QHP. Navigators are also required to conduct activities to raise awareness of an exchange.[55]

---

[51] §1311(d)(4) of ACA. In the final rule on the establishment of exchanges (77 *Federal Register* 18310, March 27, 2012) it is indicated that the rating system will be addressed in future rulemaking.

[52] HHS more specifically describes the consumer assistance functions of federally-facilitated exchanges, including partnerships, in guidance available at http://cciio.cms.gov/resources/files/FFE_Guidance_FINAL_VERSION_051612.pdf.

[53] The standard format an exchange is expected to use to present QHPs is required to include the uniform outline of coverage as established under §2715 of the PHSA (§1001 of ACA). For more information about the uniform outline of coverage, see CRS Report R42069, *Private Health Insurance Market Reforms in the Patient Protection and Affordable Care Act (ACA)*, by Annie L. Mach and Bernadette Fernandez.

[54] The final rule on exchange establishment (77 *Federal Register* 18310, March 27, 2012) does not specify the content or quantity of these outreach and education activities, but it does require that the activities must be accessible to all audiences, including to individuals with disabilities and those with limited English proficiency.

[55] §1311(i) of ACA and 77 *Federal Register* 18310, March 27, 2012.

- Include results on its website from the Secretary's survey on enrollee satisfaction with the QHPs offered through the exchange, in a manner that allows for easy comparisons of enrollee satisfaction levels.[56]

- Regularly consult with stakeholders regarding the accessibility and administration of an exchange. These stakeholders include enrollees of QHPs; individuals and entities with experience in facilitating enrollment in health insurance coverage; advocates for hard to reach populations (e.g., individuals with substance abuse problems); small businesses, large employers, and self-employed individuals; state Medicaid and CHIP agencies; federally recognized Tribes; public health experts; issuers; and health insurance agents and brokers.[57]

- Share financial information on its website, regarding: any regulatory fees or other payments required by the exchange; administrative costs of the exchange; and monies lost to waste, fraud, and abuse.[58]

- Determine the role of agents and brokers in the exchange. An exchange may allow agents and brokers to be Navigators, provided they otherwise meet the Navigator eligibility criteria.[59] An exchange may also allow agents and brokers to enroll individuals and employers in QHPs offered through an exchange if the agents and brokers meet certain requirements.[60]

Financial Management

Exchanges are responsible for financial management and are expected to be self-sustaining by 2015. They have been given authority to generate funding to support their operations; however, while the law and regulation describe this authority, neither specify how an exchange may or may not generate funding.[61] An example provided in regulation is that exchanges could charge participating issuers assessments or user fees.[62]

Exchanges are expected to play a role in collecting premiums and distributing the premiums to issuers. ACA requires exchanges to perform certain functions relating to financial oversight and integrity, including keeping an accurate accounting of all financial activities and submitting a report annually to the HHS Secretary concerning such accountings. Exchanges are also required to cooperate with investigations into the affairs of exchanges, conducted by the HHS Secretary in coordination with HHS Inspector General.[63]

---

[56] §1311(c)(4) of ACA. The survey is only for those QHPs that had more than 500 enrollees in the previous year. To date, HHS has not released any information about this survey.

[57] §1311(d)(6) of ACA.

[58] §1311(d)(7) of ACA.

[59] 77 *Federal Register* 18310, March 27, 2012.

[60] Ibid.

[61] §1311(d)(5) of ACA.

[62] 77 Federal Register 18310, March 27, 2012.

[63] §1313 of ACA.

> **ACA Risk Mitigation Programs**
>
> Exchanges are expected to deal with the potential for adverse selection. Adverse selection occurs when a large number of individuals who expect or plan for high use of health services enroll in more generous and often more expensive health plans (i.e., a woman who plans to become pregnant switches from a plan with less generous maternity benefits to a plan with more generous maternity benefits), while simultaneously individuals who expect or plan for low use of health services enroll in more modest plans, both in terms of price and benefits. Adverse selection can lead to health plans that have risk pools with a large number of high-cost individuals, which can lead to higher costs for individuals in the pool, and in extreme instances, possible dissolution of the pool due to an increasingly expensive risk pool.
>
> ACA establishes three risk programs to help mitigate the potential impact of adverse selection: reinsurance, risk corridors, and risk adjustment. The first two programs are temporary and are intended to provide some protection against risk in the short term before a full risk adjustment program can be developed. None of the programs are specific to exchanges; rather, they are tools that can be used both inside and outside the exchanges to mitigate the impact of adverse selection. For more information about ACA's risk programs, see **Appendix B**.

Federal Responsibilities for Establishment and Administration of All Exchanges

ACA requires federal agencies, primarily HHS, to oversee the exchanges, thus carrying out a number of responsibilities related to the establishment and administration of exchanges. Many of these responsibilities require federal agencies to create systems and criteria. For example, the HHS Secretary is required to develop the minimum criteria an exchange will use to certify QHPs to be offered through an exchange.[64] The HHS Secretary is also required to grant financial awards to states to be used to establish exchanges.

Federal Oversight

Federal agencies, primarily HHS, have oversight and other responsibilities for exchanges. These responsibilities not only relate to the general operation of the exchange, but they also relate to how an exchange is expected to share information and coordinate its duties with federal agencies.

It is beyond the scope of this report to detail all of the responsibilities ACA gives to federal agencies;[65] however, the following are general examples of duties required of federal agencies. Other examples are included in this report, where appropriate.

- The HHS Secretary is required to promulgate regulations relating to, among other things, setting standards for the establishment and operation of exchanges, the offering of QHPs through exchanges, and the establishment of the reinsurance and risk adjustment programs established by ACA.[66]

---

[64] These criteria are included in the final rule related to the establishment of exchanges (77 *Federal Register* 18310, March 27, 2012).

[65] For an overview of the rulemaking authority given to federal agencies under ACA, see CRS Report R42431, *Upcoming Rules Pursuant to the Patient Protection and Affordable Care Act: Fall 2011 Unified Agenda*, by Maeve P. Carey and Michelle D. Christensen.

[66] §1321(a)(1) of ACA.

- The HHS Secretary is expected to coordinate efforts between the exchange and other federal agencies (such as the Social Security Administration) to verify information collected by the exchange from applicants and related to eligibility for the exchange and other programs (e.g., premium tax credits).[67]
- The HHS Secretary is expected, through consultation with other entities (such as the National Association of Insurance Commissioners), to develop and maintain tools and set minimum standards for tools that exchanges may use to assist consumers with accessing the exchange.[68]

Federal Financial Assistance

While exchanges are expected to be self-sufficient by 2015, there is some limited federal assistance provided to states to help them as they develop their exchanges.[69] ACA requires the HHS Secretary to award planning and establishment grants to states for the purposes of activities related to establishing exchanges.[70] ACA gives the HHS Secretary the authority to determine the amount of the grants and to renew the grants if a state is making sufficient progress toward establishing an exchange. No planning and establishment grant may be awarded after December 31, 2014.[71]

Planning grants were given to 49 states and the District of Columbia.[72] These grants of up to $1 million each were intended to provide resources to states to help them conduct research and planning related to establishing exchanges. Establishment grants have also been awarded to a number of states. Level one establishment grants are annual awards to states who are still in the initial phases of developing exchanges, and level two establishment grants are multi-year awards intended to assist states that have made significant progress in implementation of exchanges. To date, 34 states and the District of Columbia have received level one grants, and two states have

---

[67] §1411(c) of ACA.

[68] §1311 of ACA.

[69] The CRS Congressional Distribution (CD) memorandum, "Patient Protection and Affordable Care Act: Health Insurance Exchange Planning and Establishment Grants" by C. Stephen Redhead and Annie L. Mach, includes a table that shows the federal grants (discussed in this section) that have been awarded to each state and the District of Columbia. The memorandum is available upon request from the memorandum's authors.

[70] §1311(a) of ACA. Some contend that the law does not contain explicit appropriation authority for the operation of federally facilitated exchanges, as §1311 only says that the Secretary may award planning and establishment grants to states. However, in regard to the federally facilitated exchange, the law does say that, "…the Secretary shall (directly or through agreement with a not-for-profit entity) establish and operate such exchange within the state and the Secretary shall take such actions as are necessary to implement such other requirements" (§1321(c)(1)(B)).

[71] All exchanges are expected to be self-sustaining by January 1, 2015. In guidance, however, HHS clarified that planning and establishment grants awarded through December 31, 2014 may be used for approved establishment activities after that date. For more information, see http://cciio.cms.gov/resources/files/Files2/11282011/exchange_q_and_a.pdf.pdf.

[72] Alaska is the only state that did not apply for a planning grant. Three states, Florida, Louisiana, and New Hampshire, have stated that they plan to return some or all of their planning grant funds. For more information about which states have received grants, see http://www.healthcare.gov/news/factsheets/2011/05/exchanges05232011a.html.

received level two grants.[73] In total, the states and the District of Columbia have received more than $856 million in establishment grants.[74]

The HHS Secretary is also required to award grants to eligible entities to help them develop and adapt technology systems to be used by an exchange to determine eligibility and process enrollment.[75] These "early innovator" grants were given to seven entities to help them design and implement the information technology infrastructure needed to operate an exchange.[76] The grants were awarded to entities that have "demonstrated their technical expertise and ability to develop these IT systems on a fast track schedule, and their willingness to share design and implementation solutions with other states."[77] The seven entities combined have received more than $249 million in early innovator grants.[78]

Coverage Offered through the Exchanges

Most private health insurance plans sold through exchanges must include a comprehensive set of benefits. The law specifies standards for the types and levels of coverage that can be offered through exchanges.

Coverage Levels and Benefits

Generally, exchange plans must (1) cover "essential health benefits" (EHBs), at a minimum; (2) limit cost-sharing, including out-of-pocket costs; and (3) provide coverage that meets one of four levels of plan generosity based on actuarial value (defined below).[79] These requirements will become effective beginning in 2014, to dovetail with the establishment of exchanges. The following discusses them in greater detail.

---

[73] The 34 states that have received a level one grant so far are: AL, AZ, AR, CA, CO, CT, DE, HI, ID, IL, IN, IA, KY, ME, MD, MA, MI, MN, MS, MO, NE, NV, NJ, NM, NY, NC, OR, PA, RI, SD, TN, VT, WA, and WV. The states that have received level two grants, to date, are Rhode Island and Washington.

[74] Center for Consumer Information and Insurance Oversight, "Affordable Insurance Exchanges: Update and Upcoming Implementation Forums," press release, May 16, 2012, http://cciio.cms.gov/resources/factsheets/affordable_insurance_exchanges.html.

[75] §1561 of ACA: §3021 of PHSA.

[76] The seven grantees are Kansas, Maryland, New York, Oklahoma, Oregon, Wisconsin, and a multi-state consortium led by the University of Massachusetts Medical School (which includes Connecticut, Maine, Massachusetts, Rhode Island, and Vermont). Three states, Kansas, Oklahoma, and Wisconsin, have since stated their intention to return some or all of the grant. For more information, see http://www.cbpp.org/files/CBPP-Analysis-on-the-Status-of-State-Exchange-Implementation.pdf.

[77] HealthCare.gov, "States Leading the Way on Implementation: HHS Awards "Early Innovator" Grants to Seven States," press release, February 16, 2011, http://www.healthcare.gov/news/factsheets/2011/02/exchanges02162011a.html.

[78] Center for Consumer Information and Insurance Oversight, "Affordable Insurance Exchanges: Update and Upcoming Implementation Forums," press release, May 16, 2012, http://cciio.cms.gov/resources/factsheets/affordable_insurance_exchanges.html.

[79] §1302(a)-(d) of ACA.

Essential Health Benefits

ACA does not explicitly list the benefits that comprise essential health benefits (EHBs). Instead, the law identifies 10 broad benefit categories which must be included in EHBs, at a minimum:

- ambulatory patient services;
- emergency services;
- hospitalization;
- maternity and newborn care;
- mental health and substance use disorder services, including behavioral health treatment;
- prescription drugs;
- rehabilitative and habilitative services and devices;
- laboratory services;
- preventive and wellness and chronic disease management; and
- pediatric services, including oral and vision care.

States may impose additional benefit mandates beyond what is required under EHBs. However, any state that requires health plans to offer benefits beyond EHBs must assume the total cost of providing those additional benefits, for all the plans, and regardless of whether or not an individual is receiving any financial assistance with premiums or cost-sharing. The state must make payments either directly to the individuals enrolled in health plans affected by the state benefit mandates, or to such plans on behalf of enrolled individuals.[80]

The bulk of the responsibility for defining EHBs is given to the HHS Secretary, who must then notify the public and provide the opportunity for comment. The HHS Secretary has certain guidelines that must be followed in developing the EHBs, including ensuring that the scope of EHBs is equal to the scope of benefits under a "typical" employer-provided health plan (as certified by the Chief Actuary of the Centers for Medicare & Medicaid Services), and that EHBs meet equity and other standards specified in the law. To assist the HHS Secretary in this determination, the law requires the Secretary of the Department of Labor (Labor) to conduct a survey of employer-provided health coverage.[81]

ACA did not specify a deadline for when the Secretary is required to define EHBs. To date, HHS has not issued regulations defining EHBs. Instead, HHS published a bulletin which stated that "EHB be defined by a benchmark plan selected by each State."[82] HHS identified four benchmark plan types that a state could use for the purpose of defining EHBs in that state:

---

[80] This applies to all exchange enrollees whose insurance is affected by additional state benefit mandates, not just those exchange enrollees eligible for premium tax credits and cost-sharing subsidies. §1311(d)(3)(B) of ACA.

[81] See "Selected Medical Benefits: A Report from the Department of Labor to the Department of Health and Human Services," Department of Labor, April 15, 2011, http://www.bls.gov/ncs/ebs/sp/selmedbensreport.pdf.

[82] "Essential Health Benefits Bulletin," Center for Consumer Information and Insurance Oversight, December 16, 2011, p.8, http://cciio.cms.gov/resources/files/Files2/12162011/essential_health_benefits_bulletin.pdf.

- one of the three largest plans in the state's small group health insurance market;[83]
- one of the three largest state employees health benefits plans;
- one of the three largest national plans offered through the Federal Employees Health Benefits Program (FEHBP); or
- the largest commercial non-Medicaid health maintenance organization in the state.

To assist states in this effort, HHS conducted studies that identified the largest plans (by enrollment) for several of the benchmark plan types listed above, and documented the prevalence of certain benefits in health plans that are currently offered.[84] HHS found that the largest national FEHBP plan, by far, is offered through Blue Cross and Blue Shield; and while small group plans vary by state, the ones with the largest enrollment generally are offered by large, commercial insurance carriers.

HHS asked states to select a benchmark plan by September 30, 2012. To date, HHS has not released information about state selections.[85]

Cost-Sharing Requirements

Cost-sharing includes deductibles and co-payments for services rendered. ACA limits the amount of cost-sharing that exchange plans generally may impose on enrolled individuals. These cost-sharing limits prohibit

- any deductible applicable to preventive health services;
- deductibles, in small group health plans, that are greater than $2,000 for self-only coverage, or $4,000 for any other coverage in 2014 (annually adjusted thereafter);[86] and
- annual cost-sharing limits that exceed existing limits specified in the tax code, relating to certain high deductible health plans.[87]

---

[83] In the final regulation on data collection to support essential health benefits standards, HHS stated that it will collect data from the insurance carriers that offer the three largest health plans (by enrollment) in the small group market within each state. The data collection is for purposes of identifying a potential "default benchmark plan" for each state. HHS intends to make publicly available the "information on the final state selections of benchmarks…as soon as possible." 77 *Federal Register* 42661, July 20, 2012.

[84] See "Essential Health Benefits: Comparing Benefits in Small Group Products and State and Federal Employee Plans," Office of the Assistant Secretary for Planning and Evaluation, December 2011, http://aspe.hhs.gov/health/reports/2011/MarketComparison/rb.shtml; "Essential Health Benefits: List of the Largest Three Small Group Products by State," Center for Consumer Information and Insurance Oversight, July 3, 2012, http://cciio.cms.gov/resources/files/largest-smgroup-products-7-2-2012.pdf.PDF; and "Frequently Asked Questions on Essential Health Benefits Bulletin," Centers for Medicare and Medicaid Services, February 17, 2012, http://cciio.cms.gov/resources/files/Files2/02172012/ehb-faq-508.pdf.

[85] State Reforum, a project of the National Academy for State Health Policy, is tracking state progress on selecting an essential health benefits benchmark plan at http://www.statereforum.org/state-progress-on-essential-health-benefits.

[86] While this provision specifically applies these deductible limits to small group health plans, § 1201 of ACA: new PHSA § 2707 also applies these limits to "group health plans" broadly.

[87] The cost-sharing limits that are part of the essential health benefits package mirror the limits applicable to high-deductible health plans (HDHPs) that qualify to be paired with health savings accounts (HSAs). For 2012, the cost-sharing limits for HSA-qualified HDHPs are $6,050 for single coverage, and $12,100 for family coverage. Given that (continued...)

Levels of Plan Generosity

Health plans that provide the essential health benefits package must tailor cost-sharing to meet one of four levels of generosity, based on actuarial value.[88] Actuarial value (AV) is a summary measure of a plan's generosity, expressed as the percentage of medical expenses estimated to be paid by the issuer for a standard population and set of allowed charges. In other words, AV reflects the relative share of cost-sharing that may be imposed. In general, the lower the AV, the greater the cost-sharing, on average.[89]

Each level of plan generosity is designated according to a precious metal and corresponds to a specific actuarial value:

Levels	Actuarial Value
Bronze	60%
Silver	70%
Gold	80%
Platinum	90%

While the term actuarial value may imply a high level of precision,

> actuarial analysis is inherently an estimation process and hence is somewhat inexact. Actuarial value estimates will vary by the data sources, projection methods, and assumptions used, and there may be a reasonable range of appropriate methods and assumptions used to develop these estimates.[90]

Given this, ACA requires the HHS Secretary to promulgate regulations regarding the determination of the levels of plan generosity. The determination will be based on a benefit package consisting of essential health benefits and a standard population. To date, HHS issued a bulletin that described its proposed definition for actuarial value and solicited comments. In the bulletin, HHS proposes to use a standard data set based on a countrywide standard population, with the option for individual states to "develop State standard populations based on State claims data."[91]

(...continued)
the existing limits are updated annually and ACA cost-sharing requirements become effective in 2014, the cost-sharing limits in 2014 will likely be different than the 2012 levels.

[88] While actuarial value (AV) is a useful measure, it is only one component that addresses the value of any given benefit package. AV, by itself, does not address other important features of coverage, such as total (dollar) value, network adequacy, and premiums.

[89] While actuarial value is calculated based on costs for an entire population, it does not mean that every person enrolled in the same plan will have the same expenses, because in any given group some people use relatively little care while others use a great deal. Given that actuarial value reflects cost-sharing, such a measure may be useful to consumers when comparing different health plans.

[90] "Critical Issues in Health Reform: Actuarial Equivalence," American Academy of Actuaries, May 2009, p. 4, available online at http://www.actuary.org/pdf/health/equivalence_may09.pdf.

[91] "Actuarial Value and Cost-Sharing Reductions Bulletin," Center for Consumer Information and Insurance Oversight, February 24, 2012, http://cciio.cms.gov/resources/files/Files2/02242012/Av-csr-bulletin.pdf, p. 5.

Exchange Health Plans

Exchanges will offer several types of health plans, as specified in statute and regulation. Exchange plans will provide a comprehensive set of covered benefits (i.e., the essential health benefits), except for stand-alone dental plans (which will have to meet a narrow set of benefit requirements). While most of these comprehensive plans will be available to any individual or employer who is qualified to enroll in exchanges (such as multi-state QHPs and CO-OP QHPs),[92] some plans will be available only to specific subpopulations (child-only QHPs and catastrophic QHPs).[93] Finally, some plans offered in exchanges may also be offered outside of exchanges.[94]

Qualified Health Plans

In general, exchanges will offer comprehensive coverage that meets the standards to be certified as "qualified health plans" (QHPs),[95] provided it meets requirements related to marketing, choice of providers, plan networks, and other features, or is recognized by each exchange through which such plan is offered.[96] In addition, all QHPs are required to comply with benefit, cost-sharing and generosity components of the essential health benefits package (described above). In addition to qualified health plans, exchanges will also offer multi-state QHPs, child-only QHPs, and CO-OP QHPs (described below).

An issuer of QHPs must be licensed and in good standing with each state in which it offers coverage; must offer at least one QHP each providing silver and gold levels of coverage; and must comply with regulations applicable to exchanges. An issuer may offer QHPs outside of exchanges as well as inside, but the premiums would have to be the same, even if the QHP is sold through an insurance agent.[97]

Multi-state Qualified Health Plans

Multi-state qualified health plans are designed to offer nationally available QHPs, so that individuals and small businesses will all have access to these plans, regardless of where they live. The Director of the Office of Personnel Management (OPM) will enter into contracts with issuers to offer at least two multi-state qualified health plans (MSQHPs) ultimately through every exchange in all the states.[98] Any individual eligible to purchase insurance through the exchange may enroll in an MSQHP. Enrollment is voluntary, and individuals may be eligible for premium credits and cost-sharing assistance.

---

[92] For more information about these plan types, see the "Multi-state Qualified Health Plans" and the "Consumer Operated and Oriented Plans" sections of this report.

[93] For more information about these plan types, see the "Child-Only Qualified Health Plans" and the "Catastrophic Plan" sections of this report.

[94] Plans that are offered both inside and outside of exchanges must charge the same premium. In addition, ACA allows the types of health plans that are currently offered in the private market to continue to be offered once the exchanges have been established, as long as those other plan types comply with applicable federal and state law.

[95] §1301 of ACA.

[96] §1311(c) of ACA.

[97] §1301(a)(1)(C)(iii) of ACA; and 77 *Federal Register* 18415, March 27, 2012.

[98] §1334 of ACA.

Each contract for an MSQHP will be for at least one year and can be automatically renewed if neither party provides notice to terminate. At least one contract will be with a nonprofit entity, and at least one contract cannot provide coverage for abortion services.[99] The OPM Director will enter into a contract with an issuer if the issuer offers the plan in at least 60% of states in the first year, at least 70% in the second year, at least 85% in the third year, and in all states thereafter.

An issuer offering a MSQHP must meet certain requirements and adhere to certain policies. For example, an issuer offering a MSQHP must meet the requirements in every state's exchange, offer a uniform benefits package in each state consisting of the essential health benefits, and comply with the minimum standards prescribed for carriers offering health benefits plans under the Federal Employees Health Benefits Program (FEHBP).[100] However, unlike other QHPs offered through an exchange, which are regulated by a state, MSQHPs will be licensed by states, but regulated by OPM. For example, OPM has the authority to certify, recertify, and decertify MSQHPs for participation in an exchange. If OPM certifies an MSQHP, the MSQHP is deemed certified to participate in every state's exchange.[101]

Child-Only Qualified Health Plans

ACA requires an issuer that offers a QHP through an exchange to also offer that plan as a "child-only plan."[102] Child-only plans will provide QHP coverage for individuals who are less than 21 years of age. The final regulation on exchanges stated that a child-only plan must be provided at the same level of coverage (bronze, silver, gold, or platinum) as a qualified health plan, as specified in the law.[103]

Consumer Operated and Oriented Plans

ACA establishes the Consumer Operated and Oriented Plan (CO-OP) program, with an intent to "foster the creation of qualified nonprofit health insurance issuers to offer qualified health plans in the individual and small group markets in the states in which the issuers are licensed to offer such plans."[104] ACA authorizes $3.4 billion for the program that the HHS Secretary will use to finance start-up and solvency loans to non-profit organizations applying to become qualified issuers.[105]

Health plans offered by a CO-OP loan recipient may be deemed certified as a CO-OP QHP; if a plan is deemed a CO-OP QHP, then an exchange must recognize the plan as eligible to participate in an exchange. CO-OP QHPs are eligible to participate in an exchange for two years and may be

---

[99] §1334(a) of ACA.

[100] OPM administers FEHBP and, among other duties, is authorized to negotiate benefit and premium levels with health plans that participate in FEHBP. For more information about OPM's role in FEHBP, see CRS Report RS21974, *Federal Employees Health Benefits Program: Available Health Insurance Options*, by Annie L. Mach.

[101] 77 *Federal Register* 18310, March 27, 2012. To date, OPM has not yet promulgated regulations related to MSQHPs.

[102] §1302(f) of ACA.

[103] 77 *Federal Register*, 18469, March 27, 2012.

[104] §1322(a)(2) of ACA.

[105] ACA appropriated $6 billion to the CO-OP program. The Department of Defense and Full-Year Continuing Appropriations Act, 2011 (P.L. 112-10) canceled $2.2 billion of the appropriations, and the Consolidated Appropriations Act, 2012 (P.L. 112-74) canceled an additional $400 million of the appropriations for the CO-OP program.

recertified every two years after that for up to 10 years following the life of any loan awarded. To be deemed certified, a CO-OP QHP must comply with the following: standards for certifying QHPs; all state-specific standards established by an exchange for QHPs operating in that state (except where those standards operate to exclude loan recipients due to being new issuers or based on characteristics that are inherent to being a CO-OP); and the standards of the CO-OP program as set forth in the law and the final rule relating to the CO-OP program.[106] CMS, or an entity designated by CMS, has the authority to deem CO-OP QHPs as certified to participate in an exchange.

CO-OP loan recipients must offer a CO-OP QHP at the silver and gold levels in every individual market exchange that serves the geographic regions in which the CO-OP loan recipient is licensed and intends to provide health care coverage. If offering at least one plan in the small group market, CO-OP loan recipients must offer a CO-OP QHP at both the silver and gold levels in each SHOP that serves the geographic regions in which the entity is offering coverage. This indicates that CO-OP QHPs will be offered in at least the individual market in every exchange that shares a geographic region with a CO-OP loan recipient.[107] Individuals who enroll in CO-OP QHPs offered through the individual market are eligible for premium tax credits and cost-sharing subsidies.

Catastrophic Plan

Issuers may offer catastrophic plans in the exchanges,[108] which will have actuarial values less than what is required to meet any of the levels of plan generosity for qualified health plans (described above). These plans are expected to have lower premiums, because they will have less generous coverage and higher cost-sharing. Catastrophic plans must

- be available only to individuals under 30 years of age, or individuals exempt from the individual mandate,[109] because they do not have access to affordable coverage or experienced a hardship;
- include coverage for "essential health benefits";
- include coverage for at least three primary care visits;
- have a deductible equal to existing cost-sharing limits specified in the tax code, relating to certain high deductible health plans[110] (the deductible will not apply to "preventive health services"[111]); and

---

[106] §1322 of ACA and 76 *Federal Register* 77392, December 13, 2011.

[107] According to the final rule on CO-OPs (76 *Federal Register* 77392, December 13, 2011), only two-thirds of plans offered by CO-OP loan recipients must be CO-OP QHPs offered in the individual and small group markets, indicating that CO-OP loan recipients may offer health plans that will not necessarily be available in the individual and small group markets, whether inside or outside an exchange (i.e., Medicare managed care plans).

[108] § 1302(e) of ACA.

[109] Beginning in 2014, ACA requires individuals to maintain health insurance, with some exceptions. For additional information about this provision, see CRS Report R41331, *Individual Mandate and Related Information Requirements under ACA*, by Janemarie Mulvey and Hinda Chaikind.

[110] The deductible for exchange catastrophic plans mirror the cost-sharing limits applicable to high-deductible health plans (HDHPs) that qualify to be paired with health savings accounts (HSAs). For 2012, the cost-sharing limits for HSA-qualified HDHPs are $6,050 for single coverage, and $12,100 for family coverage. Given that the existing limits are updated annually and the exchanges become operational in 2014, the deductible for exchange catastrophic plans in (continued...)

- be offered only through the individual health insurance market.

Stand-Alone Dental Benefits

ACA allows issuers to offer stand-alone dental benefits through the exchanges, as long as such benefits include pediatric oral services (as specified under the essential health benefits provision).[112] The final exchange regulation clarifies that stand-alone dental benefits may be offered in a plan separate from a qualified health plan, or in conjunction with a QHP, as specified in the law. Exchanges may not limit the offer of stand-alone dental benefits to only one of these two options. In other words, issuers have sole discretion regarding (1) whether they will offer stand-alone dental benefits, and (2) the form in which those benefits will be provided (separate from or in conjunction with a QHP).

Cost Assistance

To make exchange coverage more affordable, certain individuals will receive premium assistance in the form of federal tax credits.[113] (As specified in the law, the Treasury Department will send monthly payments to the insurance company which issues the health plan in which a credit recipient is enrolled, to cover all or part of that person's monthly premium).[114] Moreover, some recipients of premium credits may also receive subsidies towards cost-sharing expenses.[115] Exchanges have some responsibilities, as outlined below, in regard to determining an individual's eligibility for cost assistance and calculating the amount of cost assistance provided.

Premium Tax Credits

New federal tax credits were authorized in ACA to help low-middle income individuals pay for exchange coverage, beginning in 2014. The premium credit will be an advanceable, refundable tax credit, meaning tax filers need not wait until the end of the tax year in order to benefit from the credit (advance payments will actually go directly to the issuer),[116] and may claim the full credit amount even if they have little or no federal income tax liability.

To be eligible for a premium credit in an exchange, an individual must

- have household income[117] between 100% and 400% of the federal poverty level, with exceptions;[118]

(...continued)

2014 will likely be different than the 2012 HDHP/HSA limits.

[111] § 1001 of ACA; Section 2713 of the Public Health Service Act.

[112] §1311(d)(2)(B)(ii) of ACA.

[113] §1401 of ACA.

[114] While a premium credit recipient could choose to wait until the end of the tax year to claim the credit, as part of filing federal income taxes, the most likely scenario is for that individual to choose to receive the tax credit in the form of advanced payments, to coincide with the monthly payment of insurance premiums.

[115] §1402 of ACA.

[116] §1412(a)(3) of ACA.

[117] Household income is measured according to the current tax definition for "modified adjusted gross income" (MAGI). For a comprehensive discussion about MAGI and ACA, see CRS Report R41997, *Definition of Income in* (continued...)

- *not* be eligible for Medicaid or Medicare or other types of "minimum essential coverage"[119] (other than through the individual health insurance market);
- be enrolled in an exchange plan; and
- be part of a tax-filing unit.

The amount of the tax credit will vary from person to person: it depends on the household income of the tax filer (and dependents), the premium for the exchange plan in which the tax filer (and dependents) is (are) enrolled, and other factors. In certain instances, the credit amount may cover the entire premium and the tax filer pays nothing towards the premium. In other instances, the tax filer may be required to pay part (or all) of the premium.[120]

Exchanges are responsible for either determining an individual's eligibility for advance payment of premium credits or implementing a determination made by HHS.[121] If an exchange makes the determination, then the exchange is also responsible for calculating the amount of the credit in accordance with section 36B of the Internal Revenue Code.

Cost-Sharing Subsidies

Certain individuals who are eligible for premium credits in the exchanges will also be eligible for subsidies towards service-related cost-sharing. (According to guidance issued by HHS, the federal government will provide monthly payments to the issuer of the health plan in which the subsidy recipient is enrolled, to reduce the amount of cost-sharing that individual would be responsible for when s/he uses health services.[122]) An individual who qualifies for the premium credit *and* is enrolled in a silver plan[123] through an exchange, will also be eligible for a cost-sharing subsidy. As discussed above, total cost-sharing in exchange plans will be limited according to amounts specified in the federal tax code.[124] Given that most exchange plans will

---

(...continued)
ACA for Certain Medicaid Provisions and Premium Credits, coordinated by Janemarie Mulvey.

[118] An exception is made for lawfully present aliens with income below 100% of the FPL, who are ineligible for Medicaid for the first five years that they are lawfully present. These taxpayers will be treated as though their income is exactly 100% of FPL for purposes of the premium credit.

[119] The definition of minimum essential coverage is broad. It includes Medicare Part A, Medicaid, the State Children's Health Insurance Program (CHIP), Tricare, the TRICARE for Life program, the veteran's health care program, the Peace Corps program, a government plan (local, state, federal) including the Federal Employees Health Benefits Program (FEHBP) and any plan established by an Indian tribal government, any plan offered in the individual, small group or large group market, a grandfathered health plan, and any other health benefits coverage, such as a state health benefits risk pool, as recognized by the HHS Secretary in coordination with the Treasury Secretary.

[120] For a comprehensive discussion of the premium tax credits, including illustrative examples of possible credit amounts, see CRS Report R41137, *Health Insurance Premium Credits in the Patient Protection and Affordable Care Act (ACA)*, by Bernadette Fernandez and Thomas Gabe.

[121] See the "Eligibility for Premium Tax Credits and Cost-Sharing Subsidies" section in this report for more information.

[122] This proposed approach for implementing the cost-sharing subsidies was discussed in a bulletin issued by HHS: "Actuarial Value and Cost-Sharing Reductions Bulletin," February 24, 2012, - http://cciio.cms.gov/resources/files/Files2/02242012/Av-csr-bulletin.pdf.

[123] See previous discussion of precious metal designations for exchange plans under the section "Levels of Plan Generosity" in this report.

[124] The cost-sharing limits that are part of the essential health benefits package mirror the limits applicable to high-deductible health plans (HDHPs) that qualify to be paired with health savings accounts (HSAs). For 2012, the cost-
(continued...)

already be required to meet such limits, the cost-sharing subsidies will further reduce the total amount those individuals who qualify for the subsidies will pay for using health services.[125]

Exchanges are required to either determine an individual's eligibility for cost-sharing subsidies or implement a determination made by HHS.[126] To do this, an exchange is expected to collect and verify the information necessary to make the determination and share that information with HHS.

Interaction with Other ACA Provisions

Individual Mandate

Beginning in 2014, most individuals are required to have health insurance or potentially pay a penalty for noncompliance.[127] Generally, individuals will be required to maintain "minimum essential coverage" for themselves and their dependents.[128] Nearly all plans offered through exchanges qualify as minimum essential coverage. As follows, most individuals who have coverage through an exchange will meet the requirements of the individual mandate. Other coverage, such as employer-sponsored insurance and Medicaid, is also considered minimum essential coverage for the purpose of the individual mandate, so an individual does not have to enroll in an exchange plan to meet the requirements of the mandate.

Certain individuals will be exempt from the individual mandate. For example, some individuals will qualify for an exemption based on the affordability of coverage while others will qualify because of their religious beliefs. In screening applicants for eligibility for QHPs and IAPs, exchanges are required to determine whether an individual is exempt from the mandate and issue certificates of exemption accordingly.[129]

(...continued)

sharing limits for HSA-qualified HDHPs are $6,050 for single coverage, and $12,100 for family coverage. Given that the existing limits are updated annually and ACA cost-sharing requirements become effective in 2014, the cost-sharing limits in 2014 will likely be different than the 2012 levels.

[125] For additional information about the cost-sharing subsidies, including illustrative examples, see CRS Report R41137, *Health Insurance Premium Credits in the Patient Protection and Affordable Care Act (ACA)*, by Bernadette Fernandez and Thomas Gabe.

[126] See the "Eligibility for Premium Tax Credits and Cost-Sharing Subsidies" section in this report for more information.

[127] The constitutionality of the individual mandate has been the centerpiece of numerous legal challenges to ACA. In March of 2012, the United States Supreme Court heard arguments related to the constitutionality question, along with other legal issues. On June 28, 2012, the Court issued its decision in *National Federation of Independent Business v. Sebelius*, finding that the individual mandate in § 5000A of the Internal Revenue Code (as added by § 1501 of the Patient Protection and Affordable Care Act (ACA)), is a constitutional exercise of Congress's authority to levy taxes. For additional discussion about the Court's decision, the individual mandate, and other ACA issues, see the CRS Legal Sidebar posts under "Health and Medicine," http://www.crs.gov/analysis/legalsidebar/pages/default.aspx?source=legalSidebar.

[128] For a list of the types of coverage that qualify as "minimum essential coverage" and additional information about the individual mandate see CRS Report R41331, *Individual Mandate and Related Information Requirements under ACA*, by Janemarie Mulvey and Hinda Chaikind.

[129] In the final rule on exchange establishment (77 *Federal Register* 18310, March 27, 2012), HHS indicated that in future rulemaking it will address the process exchanges will use to provide certificates of exemption.

Employer Requirements

While employers are not required to offer health benefits to their employees, certain large employers may be subject to penalties whether or not they offer health insurance. Large employers who do *not* offer health insurance may be subject to penalties if any of their *full-time* workers enroll in exchange plans and receive premium credits. While most employers who *do* offer health benefits will meet the law's requirements, some also may be required to pay a penalty if any of their full-time workers receive a premium credit.[130]

In the latter scenario, one way that workers with an employer offer of health benefits may be eligible for premium credits is if the employer plan does not provide minimum value; that is, has an actuarial value that is less than 60%.[131] So while employers are not required to offer coverage through the exchanges, certain large employers may be subject to a penalty if they offer coverage with an actuarial value lower than a bronze-level plan and one of their full-time workers enrolls in an exchange and receives a premium credit.

Exchanges are responsible for notifying an employer if an employee has been found eligible for advance payment of premium credits or cost-sharing subsidies. The exchange must identify the employee, indicate the employee's eligibility, explain that the employer may be subject to penalty, and notify the employer of the right to appeal the determination.

Reforms to Private Health Insurance Markets

ACA includes a number of private market reforms that impose requirements on health insurance carriers and others. Such reforms relate to the offer, issuance, generosity, and pricing of health plans, among other requirements. For example, ACA requires most health plans to extend dependent coverage to children under age 26, with exception.[132] Given that health insurance carriers will be offering plans through the exchanges, ACA's private market reforms will apply to exchange plans.[133]

As discussed under the "Plan Management Responsibilities" section of this report, one of the responsibilities of exchanges will be to certify that plans meet the criteria for a qualified health plan, and, therefore, may be offered through an exchange. While the certification process will consider plan marketing requirements, provider network adequacy, and other features, as specified in the law, the market reforms are requirements imposed generally on insurance companies. Since states remain the primary regulators of health insurance, even post-ACA enactment, states would enforce ACA insurance requirements.

---

[130] For additional information about employer requirements under ACA, see CRS Report R41159, *Summary of Potential Employer Penalties Under the Patient Protection and Affordable Care Act (PPACA)*, by Janemarie Mulvey.

[131] §1401(a) of ACA; adding a new §36B(c)(2)(C) to the Internal Revenue Code.

[132] For additional information about ACA's private market reforms, see CRS Report R42069, *Private Health Insurance Market Reforms in the Patient Protection and Affordable Care Act (ACA)*, by Annie L. Mach and Bernadette Fernandez.

[133] Note that ACA does not prohibit such carriers from offering coverage outside of exchanges – see §1312 (d)(1)(A) of ACA.

Medicaid

While Medicaid is generally beyond the scope of this report, ACA's Medicaid and exchange provisions were originally designed to work in tandem with each other to provide a continuous source of subsidized coverage for low- to middle-income individuals and families, beginning in 2014. As previously discussed, exchanges are responsible for facilitating enrollment in Medicaid.

As *originally* enacted, ACA required states to expand Medicaid to certain individuals who are under age 65 with income up to 133%[134] of the federal poverty level (FPL), beginning in 2014. This reform not only expanded eligibility to a group that generally is not eligible for Medicaid (low-income childless adults), but also raised Medicaid's mandatory income eligibility level for certain existing groups to 133% of the FPL. States were required to do this mandatory expansion as a condition of receipt of Medicaid federal financial participation. Given that premium credits would be available through all state exchanges at the same time as this Medicaid expansion, the law envisioned that all individuals with income up to 400% FPL would have access to subsidized coverage, regardless of their state of residency.

On June 28, 2012, the United States Supreme Court issued its decision in *National Federation of Independent Business v. Sebelius*. The Court held that the federal government cannot terminate current Medicaid program federal matching funds if a state refuses to expand its Medicaid program to include non-elderly, non-pregnant adults under 133% of the federal poverty level. If a state accepts the new ACA Medicaid expansion funds, it must abide by the new expansion coverage rules, but, based on the Court's opinion, it appears that a state can refuse to participate in the expansion without losing any of its current federal Medicaid matching funds. All other provisions of ACA, including the entire Health Care and Education Reconciliation Act (HCERA, P.L. 111-152), remain intact. Given that some states may choose not to expand Medicaid, there is a possibility that some individuals will not have access to either Medicaid or the premium tax credits.

Regardless of whether or not a state expands its Medicaid program, the rules for coordination and facilitating enrollment between exchange plans and Medicaid will still apply. For example, an individual exchange may decide to determine eligibility for Medicaid.[135] If a person who has

---

[134] In addition, there is a 5% income disregard, so that the limit is 138% of the FPL.

[135] For more information about an individual exchange's responsibilities relating to screening individuals for Medicaid, see the "**Source:** CRS analysis of ACA (as amended) and 77 Federal Register 18310, March 27, 2012.

a. These criteria are detailed in **Table 1**.

b. The definition of minimum essential coverage is discussed in CRS Report R41331, *Individual Mandate and Related Information Requirements under ACA*, by Janemarie Mulvey and Hinda Chaikind.

c. The Personal Responsibility and Work Opportunity Reconciliation Act of 1996 (P.L. 104-193) determined that most individuals who are not citizens but are lawfully present in the United States are barred from Medicaid for the first five years that they are in the United States.

d. A description of the different tiers of coverage offered through an exchange is included in the "Coverage Levels and Benefits" section of this report.

e. The cost-sharing subsidies reduces the annual caps on out-of-pocket expenses for individuals with income between 100% and 400% FPL. Additionally, ACA requires QHP issuers to further reduce cost-sharing requirements for individuals with income between 100% and 250% FPL. For more information, see CRS Report R41137, *Health Insurance Premium Credits in the Patient Protection and Affordable Care Act (ACA)*, by Bernadette Fernandez and Thomas Gabe.

(continued...)

applied for exchange coverage is determined eligible for Medicaid, the individual exchange must enroll the person in Medicaid and share the person's information with the state Medicaid agency.

(...continued)
Eligibility for Medicaid and CHIP" section in this report.

Appendix A. Selected Exchange Implementation Dates

Table A-1. Selected Upcoming Exchange Implementation Dates

Date	Requirement
3rd Quarter, CY2012	States must specify a benchmark plan to serve as the reference plan for the essential health benefits (EHB) for coverage years 2014 and 2015.[a]
November 16, 2012	States seeking to administer all or part of their exchanges must submit a complete exchange blueprint no later than this date to be considered for exchange approval by January 1, 2013.
January 1, 2013	Each exchange must be approved to operate by HHS no later than this date in order to be operational on January 1, 2014.
October 1, 2013	Open enrollment must begin for coverage offered through an exchange for the 2014 coverage year.
January 1, 2014	Exchanges must be established and offer coverage in every state.

Source: Table prepared by CRS based on information collected from (1) ACA (P.L. 111-148, as amended); (2) 77 *Federal Register* 18310; and (3) *Draft Blueprint for Approval of Affordable State-based and State Partnership Insurance Exchanges,* at http://cciio.cms.gov/resources/files/Exchangeblueprint05162012.pdf.

a. This information was included in the Essential Health Benefits Bulletin released by HHS in December 2011. The bulletin provides information about the regulatory approach HHS intends to propose to define EHB. To date, HHS has not published regulations relating to EHB. The EHB Bulletin is available at http://cciio.cms.gov/resources/files/Files2/12162011/essential_health_benefits_bulletin.pdf.

Appendix B. Risk Mitigation Programs Under ACA

Table B-1. Description of Reinsurance, Risk Corridors, and Risk-Adjustment Provisions of ACA

	Reinsurance	Risk Corridors	Risk- Adjustment
Description	Reinsurance typically is thought of as insurance for insurers. When issuing policies, an insurer faces the risk that the premiums it collects will not be sufficient to cover its expenses and generate profit. Reinsurance shifts the risk of covering high expenses from the primary insurer to a reinsurer. ACA requires all health insurance issuers and third-party administrators of group health plans to contribute to a reinsurance program administered by a nonprofit reinsurance entity.	Risk corridors refer to a mechanism that adjusts payments to health plans according to a formula based on each plan's actual, allowed expenses in relation to a target amount. If a plan's expenses exceed a certain percentage above the target, the plan's payment is increased. Likewise, if a plan's expenses exceed a certain percentage below the target, the plan's payment is decreased. Under ACA, a QHP issuer whose gains are greater than 3% of the issuer's "projections" must remit charges to HHS, while HHS must make payments to a QHP issuer that experiences losses that are greater than 3% of the issuer's "projections."	Risk adjustment refers to a mechanism that adjusts payments to health plans to take into account the risk that each plan is bearing based on its enrollee population. Plans with enrollment of less than average risk will pay an assessment to the state. States will provide payments to plans with higher than average risk.
Objective	Provide funding to plans that enroll highest cost individuals	Limit issuer loss (and gains)	Transfer funds from lowest risk plans to highest risk plans
Goal	Offset high-cost outliers	Protect against inaccurate rate setting	Protect against adverse selection
Who Participates	Non-grandfathered individual market plans (inside and outside of exchange) are eligible for payments	Qualified Health Plans (QHPs) in the individual and small group markets (inside and outside of exchange)	Non-grandfathered individual and small group market plans (inside and outside the exchange, excluding self-insured plans)
Time Frame	Three years (2014-2016)	Three years (2014-2016)	Permanent; begins after end of benefit year 2014

Source: CRS analysis of ACA.

Author Contact Information

Bernadette Fernandez
Specialist in Health Care Financing
bfernandez@crs.loc.gov, 7-0322

Annie L. Mach
Analyst in Health Care Financing
amach@crs.loc.gov, 7-7825

www.ingramcontent.com/pod-product-compliance
Lightning Source LLC
Chambersburg PA
CBHW081244180526
45171CB00005B/541